Diets to help
ARTHRITIS

A complete dietary programme to help all those
suffering from osteo and rheumatoid arthritis.

Also in this series:

Diets to Help
ARTHRITIS

HELEN MACFARLANE

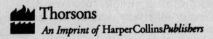
Thorsons
An Imprint of HarperCollinsPublishers

Thorsons
An Imprint of HarperCollins*Publishers*
77–85 Fulham Palace Road,
Hammersmith, London W6 8JB
1160 Battery Street,
San Francisco, California 94111–1213

First published 1979
Second edition published 1988
This edition 1994
10 9 8 7 6 5 4 3 2

A catalogue record for this book
is available from the British Library

ISBN 0 7225 2871 X

Phototypeset by Harper Phototypesetters Limited,
Northampton, England
Printed in Great Britain by
HarperCollinsManufacturing Glasgow

Contents

Introduction

One of the most persistent and long-standing theories in connection with arthritis is that the symptoms can be caused by an acid condition in the body and that this can be corrected by means of proper diet. In my own case, I have worked out a diet over the years which, along with occasional periods of physiotherapy and a sensible amount of physical exercise, has kept me free from pain and enabled me to live a normal life for the past fifteen years. Before taking these measures I had reached a point where I was almost ready for a wheelchair.

With arthritis every part and function of the body must be considered, as well as mental attitudes. It is not only a question of painful joints and muscles and weight control; it is also a question of viewing the body as a whole and realizing that arthritis is not a localized disease but a cry for help from the whole organism. In this context diet is all-important and no lasting improvement in any of the arthritic diseases can be expected if the sufferer concentrates on foods containing large proportions of white sugar and white flour and other devitalized carbohydrates, too much meat, cheese, cream, eggs, butter and frequent 'fry-ups'.

If the general guidelines in this book are followed over the long term the effect should be to reduce any excess weight and then to stabilize it to a healthy norm. This in itself will lessen stress and strain on weakened joints and on muscles and tendons which have lost their elasticity. Then, instead of a gradual and apparently inevitable loss of mobility, the way is open, if not to complete recovery, at least to improvement. This is a goal which can be aimed at day by day and the results can be surprising.

CHAPTER ONE

Why Arthritis?

Not everyone gets arthritis. Why is it, then, that some people are susceptible and others are not? Some of us seem to inherit, not arthritis itself, but a tendency towards it, and certain symptoms, which often develop early in life, are signposts pointing towards this susceptibility. Armed with the knowledge of what some of these symptoms are, it is possible to take early preventive action, as described below.

CHRONIC CATARRH

From my own experience, backed up by my reading, I now realize that chronic catarrh can be one of the first symptoms of arthritis, and this is often accompanied by so-called growing pains. Apparently catarrh is one way in which the body is attempting to give warning and to throw off the poisons generated by excess food, or by a large proportion of the wrong kinds of food, such as white flour and white sugar products. Coffee and tea, except in moderation, are also bad. Ordinary table salt is another great culprit, since it produces extreme acidity. Two substitutes can be used for this (again with moderation) – sea salt or kelp (ground seaweed).

VITAMIN A DEFICIENCY

Another likely theory, in view of the tendency of arthritics to suffer from respiratory diseases in general, is that there is a deficiency of Vitamin A in the diet or in the system. This vitamin is found in the fish liver oils and in some vegetables. It has also been found that in many instances arthritics suffer from liver disorders, so that they are not able to transform the carotene in yellow vegetables into Vitamin A.

ASSIMILATION OF CARBOHYDRATES

Many arthritics have difficulty also in assimilating carbohydrates, i.e. starches and sugars, and this process can be aided by the addition of plenty of the B vitamins, either in the diet (although this is hard to achieve owing to food processing and other factors), or in the form of food supplements such as brewer's yeast tablets.

In fact, so important are the vitamins and minerals

in sustaining health and movement, particularly for those suffering from arthritis, that a part of this book is given over to these substances and how best to obtain and use them.

RESTING THE DIGESTIVE SYSTEM

Perhaps one of the simplest and best ways of helping to restore the body to maximum health is to make a point of having one day weekly without solid foods, eating only raw fruits or soups. This gives the digestive system an opportunity to rest and to eliminate accumulated wastes.

Cutting down on meat also helps the digestive system. Remember, though, that any radical change of diet must be initiated very gradually. For instance, in the beginning meat could be omitted entirely for one or two days weekly, and in any case arthritics should not eat it more than once a day, and then in very small portions, as it is known to produce uric acid which is one of the main culprits in engendering and fostering arthritis. After a trial period meat could be alternated with other proteins, such as eggs, low-fat cheese, nuts, beans, seeds – always in moderate quantities. These meat substitutes will be discussed further on in this book.

AVOIDING DRUGS

Another problem for many arthritics who have been on drugs for many months or years, including aspirin, is of course their side-effects, and it would seem that the only way to get rid of these permanently is to get rid of the drugs themselves. This has to be done very gradually and even then there are apt to be intense reactions, including pain and mental depression. They must be tailed off very slowly, pill by pill and day by day, until the body becomes used to being deprived of them and is able to assimilate wholesome foods such as salads and raw fruits.

PERSEVERANCE

The first few weeks or even months of this new way of life, along with a sensible amount of physical activity, the gradual elimination of drugs and the working out of a diet designed to promote and restore health, may in the beginning produce unpleasant symptoms, as stated above, and will require much work and thought. But from personal experience I know that in the long run, if persevered with, it can bring countless dividends in health and happiness and a general sense of well-being, to say nothing of greatly increased mobility and a complete freedom from pain without recourse to drugs.

Like most worthwhile things these benefits do not

come of themselves. They are there waiting for those who are willing to make the effort and to persevere regardless of the inevitable lapses and setbacks.

The more obstinate and long-standing cases of osteo-arthritis might take six months or more to show any noticeable improvement, but improvement there is bound to be, particularly in general health, for anyone who has the patience and fortitude to study and abide by this or a similar corrective diet. Those with rheumatoid arthritis might also benefit from this regimen.

This is something each individual has to work out for himself, different as we are in our needs and abilities to assimilate the foods we take in. Trial and error must enter into this. There is an abundant variety of suitable foods, and a little thought and imagination can make any of them appetizing and attractive. This, or any other book or counsellor, can only set out guidelines.

OBESITY

Obesity can be and often is a problem with arthritics and there seems little doubt that this can most often be the result of eating too many calories of 'empty' and useless foods, mainly refined carbohydrates. As Rose Elliot remarks, 'there are fat eating habits and thin eating habits', and these consist largely of the way food is eaten. I myself have observed when eating out that fat people generally choose fat-producing foods, then proceed to consume them very fast in large mouthfuls at a time. In contrast, most thin people take small mouthfuls, chew slowly and carefully, often talking a lot in between times. They are not concentrating on their food as if it were the last full meal they ever expected to eat in their lives.

CHAPTER TWO

Basic Nutrition for Arthritics

Sir W. Arbuthnot Lane, one of Britain's greatest surgeons and nutritional experts, once wrote:

> There is no doubt that all forms of rheumatism are due to the disturbance of the acid-alkaline balance, and that this condition arises from faults in nutrition. Clinical experience has now amply proved that physical factors which predispose some people to rheumatism can only be successfully countered by a diet which puts all its emphasis upon alkaline-forming foods.

ACID-FORMING FOODS

Acid formation in the body can become excessive through the consuming of too great a proportion of the concentrated proteins in the diet. These acid-forming proteins are contained in foods such as meats, fish, eggs, cheese (except cottage cheese), dried beans and peas, and nuts. These should never be used in large quantities at a time and seldom more than once in any one day. For those with arthritis the bulk of the daily diet should consist of fruits and vegetables in one form or another, though occasional lapses should do no harm.

NEUTRALIZERS AND ALKALINE FOODS

Strangely enough, the so-called 'acid' fruits, which include lemon and grapefruit, have a neutralizing effect on the body acids. In addition, they aid in the removal or dispersion of minerals which have formed deposits in the cartilage of the joints. Most fresh fruits, green vegetables and dried fruits have an alkaline reaction. Spinach and rhubarb, though known to be high in oxalic acid, are rich in iron.

I am setting out below foods which tend to be alkaline in effect, hence healthy for arthritics:

- 'Acid' fruits of all kinds, though gooseberries, strawberries and blackberries should not be eaten every day, even when in season; dried fruits, including dates are always good.
- Vegetables such as celery, watercress, parsley, mint and horse radish, tomatoes, lettuce, cabbage and carrots, preferably eaten raw in small quantities.
- Cooked green peas, brussels sprouts and broccoli are all

good in rotation with one another.
- Spinach and rhubarb may be used occasionally.
- Alfalfa in tablet form and molasses are both valuable foods.

A green leaf salad daily is most essential for arthritics, but those who have not accustomed themselves to eating raw foods should eat (literally) only a leaf or two to begin with. All raw food must be chewed thoroughly and slowly and this would be a problem for those with poor teeth.

One herb which has been found to be particularly useful in combating both arthritis and migraine and other headaches is feverfew. Only a leaf or two daily is required in salads or sandwiches, but the beneficial effects do not begin to appear for at least four months. Dandelions (the smooth round-leafed kind is the least bitter), chickweed, chives, mint, borage, and many other 'weeds' and herbs are also a pleasant and beneficial addition to most salads.

VEGETABLE JUICES

Those who possess an electric juicing machine will have at hand a valuable tool for producing a good alkaline-reacting food from almost any fruit or vegetable, or a mixture of fruits *or* vegetables, not the two together. The fruits or vegetables are sliced into small pieces, then put through the machine with water added, and the resultant juice will contain all the minerals and vitamins of the fruits or vegetables with the roughage filtered out. However, this is strong stuff and to begin with only a few tablespoonsful daily should be taken, morning or night, gradually working up to a glassful. Yet food, as a general rule, should be eaten not drunk. Drinks are useful in illness or when fasting.

LIQUIDIZING RAW FOODS

This will overcome the problem of digesting raw green foods for those not accustomed to them, who have weak digestions, or have difficulty in chewing. It is also one way of using the coarse outer leaves or parts of spinach, cauliflower, lettuce, celery, cabbage or other green vegetables. These should first be washed and then chopped fairly finely with a knife or shredded by hand. The pieces are then pressed into the blender, never more than half way up, and water is added to about the quarter point or a little less.

This will be converted by the blender-liquidizer into a thick green purée composed of fine particles which are easily digested and can either be consumed as they are as a vegetable (though the taste is apt to be bitter), or added to a salad. Cottage cheese or salad dressing will disguise the strong flavour, or the purée can form the basis of a very nutritious soup. When milk is added the flavour becomes quite bland and further improvement can take place with the addition of a little kelp powder, sea salt, Marmite or other yeast spread, or soy sauce.

As in the case of raw vegetable juices, those unaccustomed to raw green foods should take only one or two tablespoonsful of this purée to begin with. The liquidizer-blender is also invaluable, of course, for many other kinds of soups, including those containing pulses such as dried beans or peas.

OTHER WAYS TO USE VEGETABLES

If a juicer or liquidizer-blender is not available, celery and the coarse leaves of vegetables can be cooked in a little water until soft, then squeezed out by hand. The resultant liquor is a healthful addition to soups, stews or gravies.

FOODS WHICH TEND TO BE ACID-FORMING

All of these foods should be used in moderation or avoided altogether by sufferers from arthritis.

All Meats, Fish and Cheeses

With the exception of cottage cheese, these should be cut down to a minimum. The goal to aim at is to have any one of these only once daily and to avoid large helpings at any time.

Eggs and Egg Products

No more than the equivalent of two or three eggs should be eaten weekly. Eggs are more easily assimilated when mixed with milk, as when scrambled.

Dried Beans, Lentils, Dried Peas and Nuts

These could be alternated with flesh foods, cheese and eggs for protein and never used in large quantities at any one time.

All White Sugar and White Flour Products

These should be used only occasionally and then sparingly on special occasions.

Alcoholic Drinks

With the possible exception of good wines (not sherry) these should not be consumed daily and never in large amounts at a time.

Deep-Fried Foods

Should never be eaten.

Strong Tea and Strong Coffee

If used several times a day these can be harmful,
particularly to the kidneys and the liver. They are acid-
producing and are likely to increase the arthritic
symptoms.

Salt

Salt (except sea salt in moderation), pickles and most
sauces are harmful to the arthritic.

The following is an excerpt from the writings of Dr
Howard Hay:

> There is no such thing as an incurable case of
> arthritis, although damage done to the joints
> previously by years of arthritis may never be
> fully corrected. The process, however, can be
> halted and a great deal of improvement enjoyed
> in every case . . . I would not touch starch or
> sugar in any form, but would live entirely on
> cooked vegetables, raw vegetable salads, fresh
> fruit and milk or buttermilk and cheese. In add-
> ition, I would suggest that you get a preparation
> of wheatgerm and take a tablespoon of this three
> times a day with honey.

Through my own experience with arthritis I find

myself disagreeing with Dr Hay in some respects. For instance I believe that a moderate amount of meat or fish once daily is preferable to consuming large quantities of milk products, including cheese, which are liable to lead to catarrh or to increase any bronchial tendencies. However, it must always be borne in mind that no two individuals are alike in their nutritional requirements and that no so-called authority can do any more than lay down general guidelines. Only through observation, trial and error over a fairly long period of time can anyone work out the diet which will bring him or her the maximum degree of health.

SET-BACKS

Dr Hay continues:

> It is not unusual to have a marked aggravation of the arthritis after you first begin changing the body's chemistry, and this is caused not by anything you are eating, but by chemicals already stored in your body that are still being precipitated. Go on in this way for a number of weeks, and you will find the condition arrested, for the pain is less and the attacks of acute arthritis less frequent and less severe.

It is known that these apparent set-backs are all part of the healing process and a sign that the body is responding. Very often a day on vegetable soup or mild fruits such as grapes or apples will put things right again.

One bonus of a diet containing plenty of fresh fruits and vegetables is that they are known to enrich the blood stream, which in turn could lead to an improvement in circulation. Poor circulation is generally associated with rheumatism and arthritis and could be one of the contributory causes.

CHAPTER THREE

Other Nutritional Guidelines

Broadly speaking, to function well the body requires proteins, fats, carbohydrates, minerals, vitamins, and various trace elements. At one time all of these and other essential elements would have been present in an ordinary 'well-balanced' diet, but the methods used today to produce, refine and/or process our foods have destroyed many (if not all in some instances) of the life-giving constituents formerly present in our diet. To replace at least some of these it has become almost a necessity to use food supplements, which will be the subject of another chapter.

PROTEINS

The amount of protein required each day per person has long been in dispute, but some of the best authorities have now come round to the view that the tendency in the developed countries has been to use quantities far in excess of the requirements of the body. This would particularly be the case for arthritics, since nearly all proteins, whether of animal or vegetable origin, are acid-producing, with the possible exception of the green-leaf proteins. Therefore the safest and best course is to limit the consumption of meat to one small portion daily, as previously stated, and when using vegetable proteins such as beans, again to take very little at a time. The same caution should be used with eggs, cheese, and other dairy products. Nuts and seeds are other good sources of protein, but here again care should be taken as to quantity.

It has now been recognized by some of those who have delved deeply into the field (not yet a 'science') of nutrition that green-leaf and whole-grain proteins can be rated as valuable foods, particularly if they are properly combined with other proteins so that 'complete' usable protein results. This will be explained in more detail in chapter 5.

FATS

Anything relating to the consumption of fats is at present an extremely controversial subject about which hardly any two 'authorities' will agree. The only safe rule for anyone is to eat only the lean parts of meat, to avoid deep-fried foods of all kinds, to avoid lard, pastries and rich puddings, to use limited quantities of butter and cream and to concentrate on the margarines which claim to be 'cholesterol-free'.

However, even some of these may be suspect because of the processing methods used in their manufacture. Moderate quantities again must be the answer to this problem.

One reason why arthritics should try to avoid the build-up of cholesterol in their veins and arteries is not only to decrease the possibility of coronaries or strokes but because this build-up will inhibit the circulation of the blood, which could be in itself one of the causes of arthritis, particularly when the muscles are affected.

Although it is as well to avoid certain fats and to consume others in limited quantities, investigators have discovered that in many primitive societies people can use large quantities of animal fats daily yet remain free from excess cholesterol until they begin to include in their diet relatively large proportions of 'civilized' food, i.e., white sugar, white flour and other devitalized carbohydrates.

ESSENTIAL FATTY ACIDS

Every fat or oil contains fatty acids, of which eight are known to be essential for the proper functioning of the body. One of the secrets of good nutrition consists in combining these eight E.F.A.s at the same time, since most proteins are deficient in at least one or two of them. Some basic rules for combining specific vegetable proteins in such a way that a complete usable protein will result are given in chapter 5.

CARBOHYDRATES

One lifelong student of nutrition who restored many sufferers to health had this to say: 'Too much food improves neither health nor efficiency, but, on the contrary, leads to premature old age and illness.' He was referring particularly to the fact that because of its poor nutritional value over-consumption of food had become a habit amongst the majority of people in the developed parts of the world, especially in the West. These bad habits are further encouraged by debasing taste buds with sugar, synthetic flavourings, salt or other seasoned foods, all in excessive quantities.

As previously stated all white sugar and white flour products have been robbed of most of their nutritive values. The best carbohydrates are found chiefly in whole-grain cereals (including wholemeal flour and brown rice), fresh fruits and vegetables, honey, molasses or dark brown sugar.

CHAPTER FOUR

Food Supplements

However carefully food is selected and combined, many essential elements may be lacking in these days of growing foods in devitalized or poisoned land and the ever-increasing tendency towards processing and fragmentation. Unless food supplements are taken regularly serious dietary deficiencies may result and these can play a large part in the onset of illnesses such as rheumatism and arthritis.

However, it should be noted that the chemical substitutes obtainable from the chemists bear no relationship to the real thing. For instance, their so-called vitamin C is a substance called ascorbic acid, quite unlike the vitamin C obtainable from the health stores, which is derived from rose hips or other naturally growing plants.

It has not yet been established exactly how many vitamins there are but a great deal has been discovered about them.

VITAMINS

Vitamin A and Carotene (or Pro-Vitamin A)

Animal foods, particularly fish liver oils, contain vitamin A; vegetable foods, particularly the yellow ones, contain carotene, though some animal foods contain both. If the diet includes nuts, whole cereals such as wholemeal bread, wheat germ, and four to eight dessertspoonsful daily of cod liver oil, there is no danger of a deficiency of these vitamins, and vitamin D will also come into this. Those with arthritis have a special need for these vitamins, and calcium, obtainable at health shops in the form of bone meal, is necessary for their assimilation.

The B Vitamins

The fact that most arthritics have difficulty in assimilating carbohydrates and consequently can suffer from chronic catarrh may point to a deficiency of the B vitamins. One of the best ways to remedy this is to take brewer's yeast tablets, beginning with two daily, with meals, for three or four weeks, then gradually increasing to six or eight daily. It is generally wise to take about three months before reaching the maximum number, otherwise indigestion may occur, in which case it is best to leave the tablets off altogether for about a week, then go back to two or three. If the body has suffered a deficiency of any specific nutrient over a long period it will not always begin to assimilate it properly over the short term.

Once the system has become used to the brewer's yeast it will be found to help the digestion, and it is also invaluable for the health of the eyes.

As well as the yeast it is advisable for those with arthritis to take supplementary vitamin B_{12} (found in liver and in some plants), which is also available in tablet form in health stores. This has been found by experiments to show remarkable results in the treatment of osteo-arthritis.

Lean meats (if not overcooked), poultry, fish and milk, dark green leafy vegetables, particularly if eaten raw, nuts and whole-grain breads or cereals, all are good sources of various B vitamins. Wheat germ, now freely available in many grocery shops as well as health stores, is rich in most of the B vitamin complex.

Vitamin C

This is contained in many fruits and vegetables, and has been found to be abnormally low in the blood of arthritics. Much has been written about experiments conducted with this vitamin. Everyone suffering from arthritis needs more than normal amounts of vitamin C every day for many reasons too technical to go into here.

If it is impracticable to eat large amounts of fruits or vegetables adequate amounts of vitamin C may be obtained from rose hip or other tablets found in health shops. These are even more effective if combined with the bioflavonoids. The bioflavanoids (vitamin P) occur under the outer skin of citrus fruits.

Most green vegetables, raw or properly cooked in a minimum amount of water or steamed, are excellent sources of vitamin C, as are many fruits.

Vitamin D

This is the so-called sunshine vitamin because it is normally absorbed through the skin in sunny weather and may be in short supply during the winter months or for house-bound people. It is found, like vitamin A, in the fish liver oils, and helps the body to assimilate other substances, particularly calcium. So many vitamins and minerals are more effective when in combination with one another.

Vitamin E

This is particularly useful in cases of muscular rheumatism (fibrositis) and will often give relief when taken in sufficient quantities over a long period of time, even with rheumatic fever and rheumatoid arthritis. Vitamin E plays a large part in assuring that all the cells of the body receive adequate oxygen, the net result being that it increases the flow of blood. It is also useful in counteracting the effects of rancid or over-processed fats and oils.

The recommended quantity to be taken to begin with is two 30 i.u. tablets or capsules twice daily after meals. Later these could be increased to 100 i.u. tablets or capsules, one after each meal. (Incidentally some of these vitamins are stated to be in mg instead of i.u.'s.) Each individual must discover by experience the amount he can best tolerate.

MINERALS

These are equally important to the health of the body as the vitamins. There are numerous minerals and trace elements required for maximum health but certain substances are so rich in them, balanced and mixed together in a way in which they can be assimilated by the body, that they deserve special mention.

Wheat Germ

As well as the invaluable vitamin E, wheat germ contains 23 known rebuilding minerals.

Sea Vegetables

The most easily obtained sea vegetable is kelp, a seaweed found in deep oceanic waters. It is brought to the land, dried, and can be purchased in powder or tablet form at health food stores. Kelp is one of the best mineral sources of iodine, easily digested and assimilated because it is combined with other compatible minerals, vitamins, trace elements, etc. The elements contained in kelp are in the exact proportions needed by the human blood stream. Incidentally, as in the case of the B vitamins, a lack of iodine in the diet can adversely affect the vision.

D. T. Quigley, M.D., has this to say in his book, *The National Malnutrition:* 'Iodine, since it has to do with increasing anti-bacterial elements in the blood, is of value in every type of rheumatic disease.'

Calcium

This is most essential for every cell of the body, particularly for the muscles. A deficiency of calcium can lead to the familiar muscle cramps, and according to Dr L. W. Cromwell in his report to the Gerontological Society of San Francisco, calcium deficiency among his patients has been found to be a cause of arthritic crippling. The regular consumption of bone meal tablets (obtainable at health stores), combined with a healthy diet, can help to prevent or eliminate muscle cramp and also to prevent or correct the crumbling or brittleness of the bones (osteoporosis) so often associated with arthritis and with elderly people.

Calcium is even more effective when taken in conjunction with wheat germ or vitamin E capsules.

It is also more effective when taken along with vitamins A and D. In fact, vitamin D is not well absorbed into the body without it.

Potassium

Potassium is a mineral of great importance to those suffering from arthritis, since it is an anti-calcification factor and will help to prevent calcium from settling in and stiffening up the joints. This calcification can be caused by a deficiency of either calcium or potassium. Foods rich in potassium are:

  most green leafy vegetables
  celery
  wheat germ
  kelp
  sesame seeds
  figs
  dark brown sugar (not the dyed variety!)
  molasses

POTASSIUM BROTH
Use young carrots with their tops, spinach leaves and stems, chopped-up celery, including leaves, parsley, cabbage and other green vegetables, as available and as fresh as possible. Chop finely, cover with water and simmer gently in a covered saucepan for about 30 minutes. Squeeze out or strain and flavour to taste.

NUTS AND SEEDS

Nuts and seeds of all kinds are good sources of protein, vitamins, minerals, trace and other elements still unknown to nutritionists. These are so packed with nourishment that they should be used with the greatest moderation. They are expensive (the seeds can be obtained at health stores), but, because of the minimal quantities required, will go far. The most usual ones are sunflower, pumpkin and sesame.

CHAPTER FIVE

Meat Savers and Substitutes

It is possible to lead a healthy life by omitting flesh foods entirely from the diet, but in view of the amount of knowledge and experience needed to carry this through successfully, for the great majority of people, particularly the elderly or infirm, any radical or sudden change of diet is not advisable.

One particular snag inherent in vegetarianism is that over the long term a vitamin B_{12} deficiency is likely to build up and this can be very serious. To offset this it would be necessary to take regularly tablets of B_{12} obtainable from health stores.

However, replacing flesh foods with vegetarian meals several times weekly would be quite practicable if it is borne in mind that a fully balanced vegetarian meal should contain 'complementary proteins', that is, two or more substances which when combined (and eaten together at the same time) will form a complete protein. Anyone interested in becoming a vegetarian would be advised to obtain books dealing specifically with this subject of complementary proteins, and with vegetarianism in general.

A few recipes using complementary proteins are given below, followed by a table showing other examples of complementary proteins. All complete proteins or complementary protein combinations contain the eight Essential Fatty Acids already referred to in chapter 3.

Baked Potatoes

If an oven is not available, or seldom used for reasons of economy, potatoes of a good shape and size may be partially cooked by boiling or steaming, cut in half, and placed under a medium grill for about half an hour. When eaten with cheese this is a complete protein meal.

Spaghetti or Macaroni Bake

1 large or 2 small onions
3 oz (75g) thin wholewheat spaghetti or macaroni
1 tin tomatoes
Grated cheese
2 tablespoonsful butter or margarine

This can be left to cook in a preset oven for two hours or a little longer while you are out and then served with a green salad or a green vegetable.

Cut the onions into thin slices lengthwise and stir-

fry in butter or margarine until they are transparent
and tender – about five minutes. Turn the onions into
a casserole, spreading them evenly over the bottom.
Break the spaghetti or macaroni into small pieces and
sprinkle them over the onions. Over these put one
medium-sized tin of tomatoes, or fresh equivalent,
then top with grated cheese, or dot small pieces over
all (avoid the processed cheese wrapped in plastic).
Cover dish and bake for about two hours in a slow
oven 275° to 300°F (135–149°C/Gas Mark 1),
according to when you wish it to be ready. This is a
complete protein dish.

Rice and Tomato Dish

½ cupful raw brown rice
2 tablespoonsful wheat germ (to complete protein)
1 cupful tomatoes
1 medium onion
sea salt
pepper
½ teaspoonful kelp powder

Bring the rice to the boil, then cook in fast boiling
water until cooked. Slice the onion thinly lengthwise
and stir-fry until transparent. When the rice is cooked
add to it the other ingredients. Put into a shallow dish,
sprinkle wholewheat breadcrumbs over the top, dab
a little butter on and heat through under a medium
grill or in the oven.

The following table gives further examples of complementary proteins:

COMPLEMENTARY VEGETABLE PROTEINS

Complementary Proteins	Proportions
Beans (dried) and any whole grains (whole wheat, oats, etc.)	1 part raw beans to 2½ parts grain.
Dried beans with cheese or other milk product.	1 part raw beans and milk, cheese, etc., according to recipe or to taste.
Dried beans or peas with brown rice.	1 part beans or peas to 4 of cooked rice.
Beans with sesame or sunflower seeds.	1 part beans to 2 of seeds.
Peanut butter or chopped peanuts with dried milk (for sandwiches)	3 parts peanuts to 1 of milk powder.
Peanut butter or peanuts and sunflower seeds (for sandwiches).	Equal quantities.

Complementary Proteins	Proportions
Potato and milk or milk product, such as cheese.	According to recipe or taste, e.g., baked potato with sprinkle of cheese when split open.
Soy flour with sesame seeds and peanut butter.	Equal quantities. Can be used as a spread (for this the soy flour is roasted until brown in a dry pan and stirred constantly over medium heat).

Small amounts of milk or milk products added to the following can greatly increase the protein quality of the dish:

   rice
   wheat
   wheat and peanuts or peanut butter
   nuts and seeds
   legumes (beans or peas)
   potatoes

Dried or liquid milk can often be added to the recipes even when this is not called for.

If these basic combinations can be borne in mind

when following recipes, a food of poor quality can be turned into a good one. For instance, when using baked beans, tinned or home made, milk should be taken at the same meal, or added to the beans, preferably low-fat powdered.

A soup made with beans or peas and milk will be a full protein meal. The same will apply if rice or whole wheat flour is used at the same meal. There are many ways of using potatoes with milk products.

TEXTURED VEGETABLE PROTEINS

Textured Vegetable Proteins (T.V.P.) are sold under various brand names both in health stores and in some grocery shops. For the most part these food products are based on the soya bean, with certain minerals and vitamins added to make a fully balanced protein food. Blended in with the bean are yeasts, spices and vegetarian flavours which produce meat-like flavours. They are a great deal cheaper than meat or fish and in some ways better, one reason being that they do not produce cholesterol in the body. They will keep indefinitely so long as they remain in the dehydrated state in which they were packaged. They can be bought in various forms, such as minced or chunky.

An analysis of one of the best-known varieties of T.V.P. shows that it contains 52 per cent vegetable protein, a little vegetable fat, and no cholesterol. For arthritics there is the added advantage that, unlike many cereals, T.V.P. contains no gluten, which so many people with arthritis cannot assimilate. This particular T.V.P. (and there is no reason to suppose that other brands are essentially different) also contains the Essential Fatty Acids the body needs as well as many valuable minerals, especially a good proportion of potassium. This mineral is particularly essential for arthritics and is often very deficient in a modern diet. These foods are also fortified with B vitamins, including B_{12}, usually in short supply in vegetarian dishes, but of very vital importance. The calorie content is relatively low compared with the other nutrients.

One word of warning, however; anyone with a goitre or suffering from hypothyroidism, or with a tendency to suffer from a sluggish thyroid or an iodine deficiency, should either avoid soya bean products or use them only occasionally. In any case, for all consumers a teaspoonful of kelp (seaweed) powder per person would be a safeguard.

Before using these textured proteins they must be hydrated, i.e., simmered or soaked in water. Directions will be on the packet. Below are a few recipes which can serve as a guide showing different methods of using these proteins to make them appetizing and interesting. There is much room for experimentation, according to the tastes and ingenuity of the user.

Baked Potatoes with T.V.P.

Baked potatoes
Minced T.V.P.
Tomatoes or onions

Have ready the baked potatoes. Soak or simmer the required amount of minced T.V.P. (about 1 tablespoonful per potato). Cut the potatoes in half and scoop out part of the middle. Mix the T.V.P. with tinned or fresh tomatoes and fill the potato shells with it. Re-heat in oven or under the grill for five to ten minutes.

Another method of using baked potatoes is to stir-fry some thinly-sliced onions, mix these with the T.V.P., and stuff the mixture into the scooped-out potatoes.

A Tasty Meal

Ham or bacon flavoured TVP
1 egg
1 tablespoonful milk
Wholewheat bread

Hydrate a small amount of T.V.P. Mix this into the egg and milk, which have been beaten well together. Dip the required number of slices of wholewheat bread into the mixture and fry both sides (or grill) until golden brown. Alternatively, place in a shallow dish and heat through under a moderate grill. Tomato ketchup or soya sauce can be used to flavour if desired.

Savoury Stew

2 oz (50g) T.V.P. chunks
2 small onions
1 cupful tinned or fresh tomatoes
1 tablespoonful brown sugar
Garlic or clove
Paprika or chilli

Hydrate the T.V.P. chunks. Slice the onions thinly lengthwise and stir-fry in a little melted butter or margarine until they are transparent. Add the tinned or fresh tomatoes, the brown sugar, a sprinkling of minced garlic or a crushed clove, a little paprika or chilli, along with some liquid from the tomatoes. Simmer for about fifteen minutes. Can be served with potatoes and/or green vegetables.

Baked Beans with T.V.P.

Ham or bacon flavoured T.V.P.
Baked beans
Wholewheat toast

Hydrate the T.V.P. and add to some heated baked

beans, using about one quarter of the amount of T.V.P. as of the beans. Serve on toast. A little tomato ketchup or soy sauce may be used if desired.

SOYA

Soya flour contains about four times as much protein as most other cereals and twice as much as pulses. When not defatted it is about 20 per cent fat. It contains no starch or sugar, but is rich in alkaline salts and essential vitamins. In southern China it is almost the only source of protein in its natural state of the whole bean. Soya flour can be used to thicken soups, sauces, gravies, etc. A small amount of soya flour added to breads, cakes, pastries or other cereal foods can greatly improve their food value. One disadvantage is that it does not keep well and needs to be used up within two or three months of purchase.

Soya Savoury

Soya flour
Mashed potato
Onion
Chives, parsley and other herbs

Using one tablespoonful of soya flour to three of mashed potato, blend together. Flavour with onion, chopped chives, parsley or other herbs and put into a greased pie dish. Heat through in oven or under grill until slightly browned.

Soya Milk

Use three tablespoonsful of soya flour (preferably defatted) to ½ pint (275ml) of water. Whisk well together, or put into blender, and use as milk. If the flour is not defatted it can be quite rich and should not be consumed in large quantities nor with great frequency.

Ready-made soya milk is available from most health food shops and from many supermarkets.

Soya Cheese

1 qt (1 litre) soya milk
¾ tablespoonful fresh lemon juice

Bring the soya milk to the boil. As it begins to rise, pour in the fresh lemon juice. Let stand until cold. Then strain through muslin, squeeze out all moisture and use as cottage cheese. Flavour to taste.

Whey – the liquid whey remaining after the making of the cheese – is a very valuable food. (If ordinary milk is used instead of a soya milk, cottage cheese can be made by using the above method.) The whey is the plasma part of the milk, i.e., the milk modified by the lactic acid culture. It contains much of the sugar and salts of the milk and also has an antibiotic reaction.

Tofu

Tofu is a very versatile soya product, in consistencies ranging from creamy to rubbery. It can be fried, chopped up in salads, or added to soups and desserts. It is available from. health food shops and some supermarkets.

LEGUMES (DRIED BEANS, PEAS, LENTILS, PEANUTS)

These are all deficient in one or two of the essential amino acids which the body needs to make up a complete usable protein. The table on page 40 lists complementary foods which can be added to make up the deficiencies.

All proteins should be consumed in very moderate amounts by those with arthritis. I think it is safe to say, for instance, that three or four tablespoonsful of dried legumes will be ample at any one meal for anyone getting on in years or unable for any reason to take a lot of strenuous physical exercise. Legumes of any sort are apt to be 'clogging' foods when used too frequently or in large helpings at a time. Those with arthritis would be well advised to use them only once or at most twice weekly. If surplus amounts are soaked and cooked they can be put into the freezer or freezing compartment of the refrigerator for future use. Some sample recipes follow:

Bean Stew with Dumplings

(This combination provides a complete usable protein)

1 small cupful beans (soaked overnight)
1 medium onion
1 small parsnip (optional)
1 teaspoonful cooking oil or fat
2 small carrots
Vegetable stock

DUMPLINGS
6 oz (175g) wholemeal self-raising flour
1 tablespoonful butter or margarine

Slice the onion lengthwise and brown in fat. Add to a cupful of vegetable stock. Scrub the carrots and cut into thin rings; cut the parsnip into three or four strips lengthwise, then into inch-long pieces. Add the vegetables to the stock mixture and simmer until the beans are soft, adding extra water or stock as necessary. Add vegetable or yeast extract for flavour.

DUMPLINGS
Rub the butter or margarine into the flour. Moisten

sufficiently with cold water so that the dough can be shaped into small balls. Drop these into the stewing pan, cover, and simmer for the last half-hour of cooking.

Bean Loaf

Cooked haricot or other beans
Grated cheese
Grated onion
Wholewheat breadcrumbs
Salt and pepper

Put the beans through a meat grinder, sieve, or blend with a little liquid, or mash them. Add one quarter the amount of grated cheese, a little grated onion, and enough wholewheat breadcrumbs to make the mixture into a loaf. Season to taste. Bake in a moderate oven, basting occasionally with a little fat. This may also be put into a shallow dish and heated through under a moderate grill.

Vegetable Casserole

¼ cupful dried beans – pre-soaked and cooked
¼ lb (100g) fresh green beans, sliced thinly
½ teaspoonful chilli powder (or less: this is very strong)
1 cupful tinned or frozen corn kernels

2 tablespoonsful grated cheese
½ cupful sliced tomatoes, fresh or tinned
A little salt
Soya sauce

Mix together the cooked beans, corn kernels, soy sauce, and other seasonings. Into a greased casserole place alternate layers of these and the other ingredients, adding the cheese last. Bake in a moderate oven for about 30 minutes. Basil and sage (sprinklings only) may be added instead of chilli if preferred. Beans and cheese make up a complementary protein. (Soya sauce is available in most grocery shops.)

Bean Meal

1 cupful haricot or kidney beans, soaked overnight
1 medium onion
1 medium carrot
Garlic
1 teaspoonful sea salt
1 teaspoonful thyme
2 tablespoonsful dessicated coconut
Milk or cream

Using the water in which the beans were soaking, add the sliced onion, sliced carrot, a crushed garlic clove or a sprinkle of minced dried garlic (sold in jars), sea salt and thyme. Let all these cook together over a low heat until the beans are tender. This will be one and a half to two hours, depending on the beans. While the mixture is still hot, stir in the desiccated coconut which has been well blended with a little milk or cream.

While the bean mixture is cooking prepare and cook brown rice or potatoes to go with it. If potatoes are used they should be mashed, using a little milk. Either rice or milk-potatoes will make a complementary protein with the beans.

CHAPTER SIX

Meat and Fish Dishes

It is generally accepted that both meat and fish are acid-producing, so that the wise course for arthritics would be to use them no more than once each day, and then in small or moderate helpings. There is also the consideration that much of the meat sold today can harbour residues such as hormones, antibiotics and other substances which can be harmful over the long term. This would apply particularly to animals or birds raised in confined spaces, such as calves, pigs and battery hens.

Fish is more easily digested than meat and less likely to be contaminated. It is also a good source of vitamins A and D, which are so important for arthritics.

MEAT RECIPES

Liver and Apples

4 slices liver
1½ tablespoonsful melted butter
1 small tart apple, sliced and peeled
1 tablespoonful wheat germ
Pinch of powdered thyme
Sea salt to taste

Mix together the thyme, salt and wheat germ. Dip the liver in the melted butter and sprinkle over it the wheat germ mixture. Brown in the fat on both sides. Leave in the pan and cover with the apple. Cover and cook over low heat for about 15 minutes. Liver is a good source of minerals and B vitamins.
(The above recipe is reproduced courtesy of Prevention *magazine.)*

Baked Chicken Legs

2 chicken legs
2 slices bacon
1 small carrot
1 small onion (thinly sliced)
1 tablespoonful sherry
1 cupful vegetable or other stock
Pinch of mixed herbs
Sea salt and pepper

Remove the meat from the chicken legs and put it with the bacon into a thick-bottomed saucepan. Add the rest of the ingredients except the sherry and simmer until the meat is tender. Add the sherry and serve.

Lamb or Mutton Stew

1 lb (450g) neck or breast of lamb
1 medium onion, cut thinly
3 medium potatoes
2 or 3 medium tomatoes
2 or 3 large slices of vegetable marrow
3 tablespoonsful raw rice
Salt and pepper

Remove the skin and superfluous fat from the meat and cut it into small pieces. Put it into a saucepan, cover with water and bring it slowly to the boil. Remove scum, add the vegetables and again bring to the boil. Cover the pan and simmer very gently for about half an hour, then sprinkle in the rice and cook slowly for another half hour, or until the meat and rice are cooked.

Sweet and Sour Beef

2 cupsful cooked beef (cut into cubes)
1 tablespoonful melted butter
2 tablespoonsful flour

1 onion, cut into thin strips
½ cupful brown sugar
½ teaspoonful dry mustard
3 tablespoonsful of cider-apple vinegar
Cooked rice, preferably brown

Stir-fry the onions in the hot fat until they are
transparent. Brown the meat slightly. Remove both
from the pan. Mix the flour into a paste with a little
cold water. Add to the fat in the frying pan. Stir
constantly until brown, adding more fat if necessary.
Put all the ingredients into a saucepan, cover with
water and simmer for about half an hour. To serve
pour over hot fluffy rice. Less meat may be used, in
which case it would be necessary to vary quantities
of other ingredients accordingly.

FISH RECIPES

Cooked Cod or Haddock with Cheese

About ½ lb (225g) or less of cooked fish (broken
    into flakes, skin and bones removed)
2 tablespoonsful butter
2–3 tablespoonsful grated cheese
¼ cupful water
1 tablespoonful flour
1 cupful milk
Breadcrumbs
Salt and pepper

Melt the butter in a saucepan, add the flour and blend well. Stir in the water, bring to the boil, stirring constantly. Simmer for five minutes. Add the milk, fish, cheese and seasoning. Turn the mixture into a shallow pan or dish which will go under the grill. Cover with fine breadcrumbs, scatter a few pieces of butter or margarine over the top and brown under a medium grill, watching to see that it does not burn or dry up. Salmon or other white fish can also be cooked in this way.

Steamed Fish

1 medium potato per person
1 medium carrot per person
Fish fillets, fresh or frozen
Peas
1 medium onion
Salt and pepper

Peel the potatoes and cut them into thin slices. Cut the carrots into thin rounds. Cook the potatoes and carrots together in just enough water to cover them. Add the peas. Cut the onion lengthwise into thin slices, and stir-fry in a little butter.

When the onion is almost soft, set it with the fish in a pan or plate on top of the saucepan containing the potatoes and other vegetables, or other vessel containing boiling water.

Prepare Tomato–Soya Sauce (see p.60) and pour it over the fish and onions.

Creamed Fish

Left-over cooked fish may be heated between two
plates over steam, then served with brown sauce,
plain or with parsley or other herbs. See also chapter
7 for ideas.

Fish Cakes

Cooked fish (skin and bones removed)
Mashed potato
1 tablespoonful chopped parsley
Salt and pepper

Mix the fish with the mashed potato and a little milk
into a stiff consistency. Add the salt and pepper and
parsley. Form the mixture into cakes and brown in hot
fat. Any surplus can be wrapped in grease-proof paper
and put into freezer or freezing compartment until
wanted.

N.B. A little onion which has been cooked by stir-frying
will add zest to any steamed or boiled fish or meat. Stir-
frying is a Chinese way of cooking which retains all
the goodness of the vegetables. It means using a
medium heat and stirring the vegetables constantly in
enough fat to coat them to the point where they are
crisp and their flavour is at its height. They should not
taste raw and they should not be brown.

CHAPTER SEVEN

Sauces and Marinades

SAUCES

Tomato Sauce

1 cupful chopped tomatoes, fresh or tinned
1 small onion
2 tablespoonsful melted butter or margarine
1 teaspoonful bayleaf powder
1 dessertspoonful cider vinegar
1 tablespoonful flour
Sea salt and pepper to taste

Put the finely-sliced or chopped onion and all the other ingredients except the flour and butter into a saucepan and boil till tender. Rub the mixture through a sieve. Stir the flour into the melted fat, add a little milk or water and bring to boil, stirring constantly. Add the tomato mixture very gradually and bring to boil, stirring all the time.

Quick Tomato-Soya Sauce

   1 dessertspoonful wholewheat flour or semolina
   ½ cup water or milk
   1 tablespoonful tomato ketchup
   1 teaspoonful soya sauce

If flour is used mix this with a little of the liquid into a smooth paste, add the remainder of the liquid and heat to boiling point over a medium fire, stirring constantly. For semolina sprinkle this over the water and milk and bring to boil, stirring all the time. If the mixture is too thick a little milk can be added as it heats. When the right consistency is reached add one tablespoonful of tomato ketchup and one teaspoonful of soya sauce.

Brown Sauce Helene

   1 small teaspoonful dry mustard
   1 large tablespoonful brown sugar
   2 teaspoonsful cider vinegar
   1 tablespoonful flour
   1 cupful water
   Handful of sultanas
   Little stewed apple
   Sprinkling of powdered bay leaf
   Sea salt

Mix well together all the dry ingredients (not the fruit, which can be optional). To these add the vinegar and water, and fruit, if used. Bring slowly to boil, stirring all the time until slightly thickened. Use for gammon or fish.

Curry Sauce

    2 oz (50g) butter or margarine
    2 tablespoonsful flour
    1 cupful cold milk or water
    1 to 3 tablespoonsful curry powder (according to taste)
    2 tablespoonsful tomato ketchup
    2 tablespoonsful desiccated coconut
    1 small onion, chopped finely
    2 tablespoonsful chopped chutney
    1 finely chopped apple (peeled and cored)
    2 or 3 tablespoonsful soaked sultanas (optional)
    Pinch of cayenne pepper
    ½ clove garlic

Heat the onion in the melted fat over a medium heat, stirring constantly until transparent. Add the curry powder, stirring well in. Mix the flour into a smooth paste with a little of the cold milk or water, add this alternately with the rest of the liquid to the fat-onion-curry mixture, blending well together over a slow heat. Stir in the tomato ketchup. Add the chutney, chopped apple and coconut and other ingredients if used. Simmer slowly over a low heat for about 15 minutes, stirring frequently.

Any surplus sauce can be stored in a covered jar in the refrigerator for two to four days, and thinned down with cold milk or water before reheating if necessary.

Tartare Sauce

    1 tablespoonful Worcester Sauce
    1 tablespoonful cider vinegar
    1 tablespoonful lemon juice
    1–2 cupsful water
    Salt

Put all the ingredients into a bowl. Set the bowl into a pan of hot water to heat the ingredients through.

Black Butter Sauce

    4 tablespoonsful butter or margarine
    1 dessertspoonful cider vinegar
    1 dessertspoonful chopped parsley
    Salt and pepper

Brown the fat in a saucepan and when it has cooled slightly add the vinegar, then reheat very slowly but do not boil. Add parsley and seasoning.

MARINADES

Marinades are useful for softening tough meats or imparting flavour to uninteresting fish. These can be soaked in the marinade for about half an hour before being cooked.

Simple Marinade

2 tablespoonsful vegetable oil
1 tablespoonful cider vinegar or lemon juice
Chopped onion
Chopped chives, parsley or other herbs
Red or white wine (optional)
Redcurrant jelly (optional)

Mix all the ingredients together. Score the meat or fish with a sharp knife, then add it to the marinade. Increase the amount of the marinade in the above proportions if required.

CHAPTER EIGHT

Salads, Soups and Sandwiches

SALADS

A good salad can provide a well-balanced and highly palatable meal, given a little forethought and imagination, and it need not be expensive, even in winter time. The variations are infinite. However, for those not used to eating raw foods it is wise to begin with to avoid too many mixtures. Start with about one teaspoonful of one raw green vegetable, perhaps parsley, and combine it with baked or steamed potato. After a few days another raw food could be added, say a little grated carrot. In all cases salads must be very thoroughly masticated if they are to be properly digested and they should never be eaten in a hurry.

Lettuce may be used with the leaves whole or shredded. Raw cabbage is a good substitute for lettuce, which is so often priced above its food value in the shops. Cabbage is fairly easy to digest if it is finely chopped or grated and eaten in small quantities at a time.

Suggested Combinations for Salads

Orange, dates, and nuts (only one or two nuts
per person)

Orange, dates and sunflower or pumpkin seeds

Raw, chopped apple with two or three nuts,
lettuce and cucumber

Celery, apple, nuts or seeds, with cheese

Pineapple and cream or cottage cheese

Raw carrot with sultanas, apple and dates

Raw carrot with sultanas and bananas

Raw carrot and raw cabbage with sultanas and
dates

These are only a few of the many combinations which
can be used to make salads which are palatable,
nutritious, and easily put together. Any of these could
be served with cottage cheese, which is an excellent
protein food.

A Basic Salad Dressing

3 tablespoonsful olive or other vegetable oil

1 tablespoonful cider vinegar

2 teaspoonsful brown sugar

1 tablespoonful milk

Shake all the ingredients well (best done in a jar). This
dressing will keep indefinitely. The proportions can be
altered according to taste.

SOUPS

Properly made and well-balanced soups can be a great standby, and can often be a meal in themselves, particularly in times of unusual stress, or when one is suffering from colds or other minor ailments, or recovering from more serious setbacks. They are a special boon to the elderly and others who are alone or handicapped. Any soup left over from the whole recipe can be stored for two or three days in a jar in the refrigerator. This is a saving on time, energy, and fuel. A good vegetable stock can be used as a base for many soups.

Vegetable Stock

  1 cupful carrots, shredded or diced
  1 cupful celery, leaves and all, finely diced
  1 cupful any other vegetable or vegetables (beet tops, turnip tops, and parsley are particularly nutritious)

This stock can in fact be made with whatever vegetables are available, in any combinations, both roots and tops. It can be flavoured with herbs such as marjoram, bay leaves, thyme, tied together with cotton or put into a muslin bag so that they can be withdrawn when the soup is ready for the table.

Using, if available, a stainless steel or enamel rather than an aluminium pan, put in the vegetables and add water to cover and an inch or two more. Put on the lid and cook slowly for about half an hour. Strain, squeeze the juice from the pulp and store in the refrigerator or cold larder any amount not being used immediately.

Legume Soups

All bean or pea (legume) soups if eaten with cheese or milk will provide a complete protein dish. Legumes and rice (preferably brown), a tablespoonful of wheat germ or unprocessed wheat bran to a serving, accompanied by wholewheat bread will provide a well-balanced protein meal. Sesame or sunflower seeds when eaten at the same meal as legumes also make a complete protein, equal in quality to beef steak.

The following is a useful guide for compatible herbs and vegetables:

For celery soup – nutmeg or dill
For pulses (lentils, split peas, etc.) – rosemary, marjoram, mint, parsley, thyme
For onion soup – sage
For potato soup – chives, mint, parsley, caraway seeds, nutmeg
For tomato soup – basil, marjoram, chives, mace

Quick Lentil Soup

½ cup dry lentils
Vegetable oil or butter
1 small onion, cut into thin lengthwise strips
1 carrot, cut into thin lengthwise strips
½ teaspoonful thyme and/or marjoram
1½ cupsful vegetable stock or water seasoned with
  a little Marmite and soy sauce
½ cupful tomatoes, fresh or tinned
Salt and pepper to taste

Precook the lentils. Brown the onions and carrots in a small amount of vegetable oil or butter, then add the herbs. Heat the remaining ingredients together, then add a little chopped parsley, and if desired two or three tablespoonsful of sherry. If grated cheese (about two tablespoonsful per person) is added to the soup you have a full protein meal.

Cream of Bean Soup

Tinned baked beans
Water
Milk

Put the beans through a sieve or liquidizer–blender with a little water added. Turn into a saucepan and heat through slowly, adding a little milk at a time to required amount, but not allowing it to boil. This can be served with buttered wholewheat toast.

Dumplings

Dumplings added to vegetable soups will in many cases make a complete protein and produce a better balanced meal. This can be an alternative to wholewheat bread or toast.

BASIC DUMPLING RECIPE

1½ cupsful wholewheat flour
2 level tablespoonsful vegetable fat
1 teaspoonful baking powder
A little salt

Rub the fat well into the flour until the mixture is of breadcrumb consistency. Add herbs, if desired, and enough water to make a soft but not too sticky dough. Flour hands well and form the dough into small balls. Drop them into the simmering soup or hot water half an hour before serving.

SANDWICHES AND SPREADS

My study of articles on nutrition and my own personal experience convince me that all cereal products should be consumed in moderate quantities by those suffering from arthritis, bread, preferably whole wheat, being limited to two or three rounds daily. One of the reasons for this is that, with a few exceptions, cereals contain gluten, which many arthritics have difficulty in assimilating. Another is, of course, the likelihood of obesity if they are eaten in large quantities, when they also inhibit the appetite for the more healing foods such as fruits and vegetables. The following suggestions might be useful for special occasions.

Peanut Butter

By itself this is not a complete usable protein. To make a completely usable protein sandwich use whole-wheat bread and one of the following combinations:

Peanut butter mixed with just under one part of dried skim milk to two of peanut butter.

Mashed banana can be added to the above, along with a little sharp-tasting jelly, such as redcurrant. Spread on top of the peanut butter mixture it gives it a pleasant tang.

As above, without the mashed banana.

Two parts of peanut butter to one of wheat germ instead of powdered milk.

Split a banana in half, lengthwise. Mix peanut butter with powdered milk and spread this over one half. Put the two parts together again, dip into orange juice and roll in wheat germ. This makes a well-balanced protein meal.

Peanut butter with chopped dates, mashed banana and a little wheat germ or powdered milk.

As above with a little mashed avocado pear.

Peanut butter with cottage cheese is a good protein.

CHAPTER NINE

Desserts and Confections

Stewed Apples with Dates

½ lb (225g) cooking apples
Dates
Egg white or cream (optional)

Cook the prepared apples and a handful of dates together very slowly in a little water until the apples are fluffy. Serve hot or cold with cream or yogurt.

When cool this dessert can be made more interesting by folding in egg white, beaten stiff, or whipped cream.

Alternatively, after cooking, pour into a shallow dish or pan, top with wheat germ or a little quick oats, a few dabs of butter and a little dark brown sugar. Heat this under a low grill for 10–15 minutes. Cornflakes or other dry cereal can also be used for topping.

Yogurt Compote

1 cupful yogurt
1 dessertspoonful honey
3 tablespoonsful desiccated coconut
½ cupful soaked dried apricots or sliced fresh ones
½ cupful grated apple
A little almond extract
2-3 tablespoonsful chopped or ground nuts

Blend together the yogurt and honey, then add the remaining ingredients. This is quick and easy to prepare and useful in suitable quantities for unexpected guests.

Quick Crust

2 cupsful granola
½ cupful wholewheat flour
2 tablespoonsful powdered milk
¼ cupful cooking oil or melted margarine

Mix the dry ingredients together and stir the oil well in, very gradually, making sure the mixture does not become too moist. Spread over the bottom of a pie dish and put filling on top, or in the case of a fruit pie spread the granola crust on top. Heat through in a moderate oven or under a moderate grill.

Cheese Crust

½ cupful mild cheese (grated)
1 cupful wholewheat flour (or white and wholewheat mixed)
½ teaspoonful salt
1 tablespoonful water

Mix together the cheese and flour. Add the salt. Drop
in the water and stir or cut this into the mixture until
it is all blended, adding a little more water drop by
drop if necessary. When the mixture can be handled
roll it out on a floured board and use as desired.

Crispy Porcupines

1 egg
½ cupful brown sugar
1 teaspoonful vanilla essence
3 cupsful puffed wheat or rice previously crisped in
   oven or under grill if they have gone limp
Desiccated coconut
1½ cupsful chopped dates
2 tablespoonsful melted butter or margarine or
   cooking oil

Combine the beaten egg, sugar, dates and vanilla.
Cook for about 15 minutes over a medium heat,
stirring constantly to prevent sticking. Cool slightly,

then add the oil and puffed rice or wheat. Mix well. Shape into small balls. Sprinkle the coconut on to a board and roll the balls in it. These sweets will keep indefinitely in the freezing compartment or freezer.

No-Bake Fruit Bars

    1 cupful seedless raisins
    1 cupful assorted dried fruit
    ¼ cupful digestive or other biscuit crumbs
    ½ cupful almonds
    ¼ cupful dried milk powder
    3–4 tablespoonsful molasses
    Desiccated coconut (optional)

Chop the fruit and nuts. Combine with the milk powder and biscuit crumbs, then add the molasses very gradually and mix well. Shape into logs about an inch round and long enough to handle with ease. (These will be easier to handle if rolled in coconut or ground nuts.) Wrap in foil or a plastic bag to store or slice into one inch bars and serve immediately. Will keep best in freezing compartment or deep freezer.
(The above recipe is reproduced courtesy of Prevention *magazine.)*

Wheat Germ Sweet

    1 tablespoonful black molasses

1 teaspoonful honey
½ cupful dry skim milk powder
1 cupful wheat germ
Ground nuts

Heat the molasses and honey together in a bowl set over hot water. Add the milk powder and wheat germ. Knead together on a board, adding ground nuts or nuts cut into small pieces. Form into small pieces and roll in ground nuts. These snacks are packed full of good nourishment and can be kept indefinitely in a freezing compartment or deep freezer. If desired desiccated coconut may be used in place of the ground nuts to roll the balls in.

A Summing-Up

If the whole of this book were summarized in a few words, what would emerge would be something along these lines:

1 Everyone with arthritis should be more concerned with quality rather than quantity of food.
2 The right kinds of food eaten in moderate quantities will not produce obesity, which is so often one of the greatest handicaps for those attempting to cope with arthritis in any of its forms.
3 White flour and white sugar products should be consumed in very limited quantities.
4 It is helpful to eat a little fresh fruit or raw salad *before* each meal.
5 Proteins of any sort should be consumed sparingly.
6 The bulk of the diet should consist of vegetables (raw or cooked), including potatoes cooked in their jackets, fruits, moderate quantities of whole cereals, some protein foods, including nuts and seeds, such as sunflower. Nuts and seeds are valuable sources of trace elements, as well as vitamins, minerals and protein.

Index